Crystal

Vision

Working with Guides, Angels and Masters:

we are never alone.

Vol 2

Extract from the original book,

'A Glimpse in a Transient Zone'

Jo Eaton.

Copyright.

Disclaimer.

The author of this book does not dispense medical advice or prescribe the use of any technique as a form of treatment for physical or medical problems without the advice of a physician, either directly or indirectly. The intent of the author is only to offer information of a general nature to help you in your quest for emotional and spiritual well-being. In the event you use any of the information in this book for yourself, which Is your constitutional right, the author and the publisher assume no responsibility for your actions.

In order to protect identity, I have changed the names of some of the characters within many of the stories.

CONTENTS

Chapter 1.

We Are Never Alone.

Sometimes, I am aware that my life appears disjointed, almost out of kilter, with outward distractions taking my time, when I then return to my old negative habits of self-doubt, or being driven by ego. I become frustrated in the realisation that I am not doing what I need to do. I am not in harmony with Spirit.

It is possible to realign with your life's purpose through meditation and by allowing Spirit to guide you. Invariably, there becomes subtle changes and opportunities appearing to assist you on your chosen path, with vitality and the enthusiasm for life increasing, almost acting as confirmation you are back on track.

Throughout history, there have been gifted avatars resonating at such high vibrations, such as Krishna, Jesus, Mohammed and Buddha, with their inspirational teachings. We must all aspire to raise our energy vibrations for the good of all, as we all occupy this infinite space in the ever-changing universe.

As we are infinite and interconnected, it is for this reason we need to be kind and generous to each other, to be grateful for what we have in this life and to stay focused on our dreams and desires, as there is an immeasurable supply of energy in the universe for our aspirations to materialise. We just need to learn to eradicate our doubts and fears and be passionate about our endeavours, for the short time we are here, while remembering we are never alone but connected to Source, living out our destiny.

I have actually experimented with my husband with this certain method, as we have had an healing session together, whether it was on one of us, or when sending distant healing to someone else. We always work in silence, then after the healing session, we compare notes of our experiences as to whom attended the healing session and what instruction or method had taken place. Invariably, our experiences are almost identical, with not only the same Masters or guides in attendance, but sometimes various other helpers too, the treatment being similar and also the advice of further follow-up sessions. This experience just reinforces our belief of the unlimited amount of assistance we each have at our disposal, if only we ask for help.

Many years ago, I was fortunate enough to meet a divine avatar from India, named Mother Meera. Although she has many followers in India, she has an ashram in Germany and travels far to extend her blessings. I attended a meeting of several hundred people in London, where I received her blessing with the placing of hands on my head, while looking deep into my eyes for several seconds. The intensity of light, through her grace and touch was memorable. There was a tremendous energy within the room, even though the actual ceremony was performed in total silence.

Mother Meera teaches us to tame our ego, in order to become aware of our highest self, then through meditation and contact with God, we are able to create and manifest into our life, all that we desire. When asked if she wanted to start a new religion, she replied,

"No, the divine is the sea. All religions are rivers leading to the sea. Some rivers wind a great deal. Why not go to the sea directly?"

I have always known there are many ways to God and yet Mother Meera's analogy is so apt. The moment she took my head into her hands and gazed into my eyes, there was such a spiritual connection of entering a divine world.

This experience endorsed my own feelings and understanding when I was just seven years of age and the realisation it is so much better for me to have a 'direct line' to God, rather than talking through other beings. I believe it is more important for me to make a personal effort to communicate on a spiritual level. This may be achieved through meditation, holding onto the silence between your words and thoughts, and with practice you are able to connect with the God-force, to 'go to the sea directly', as Mother Meera advised.

Although I attended church until I was a teenager, I became disillusioned with religion whereby the Vicar was chanting away but not making much sense to me. It was as if the congregation were very proud to be able to quickly chant several verses from memory, during the ceremony, without giving much thought to what they were saying. It was at this time when I made the decision to take the matter into my own hands and to be responsible for my own communications in prayer and meditations. From the age of eight, I already had turned to a 'direct line', one I could trust and even to this day, nothing can never dissuade me to use any other method. It serves me very well.

I am not a Roman Catholic and yet a friend once told me, if ever I mislaid anything, then I need to request the help of St. Anthony to help find the item. Mike and I have followed this advice on numerous occasions and we have always found the missing article, almost immediately. It is amazing how this works and I do not fully understand it, but I just follow the advice. It is reassuring to know we have guides, angels and helpers around us, if only we take the time to acknowledge the fact and request their assistance from time to time because all is well.

It is a pity that many people are not aware of such support and advice since it is available to all and it is so comforting to have the reassurance, to know you are not alone. It diminishes or even dissolves any fears you may hold.

Over the years, in my experience, this multisensory experience has intensified, where I am now aware of several guides, all experts in specialist areas, all loving and offering support whenever you request their assistance. It becomes quite a party at times. When you ask for help and guidance, it may not arrive instantly, or in a way you imagined, but you are always heard and there will always be some sort of response. 'Ask and it is given'.

It is important to keep in regular contact with your guides either through prayer to Source, meditation, communicating with the universe or telepathy. Whichever is your preferred method, this deeply spiritual connection is important for your wellbeing, in order to keep you strong and connected to Source. However, we must still have fun and retain our sense of humour on our journey. I remember in the early days of communicating with one of my guides, I was told life should be a fun journey on our way home.

As I have commented earlier, I have been aware of my helpers and spiritual guides for many years and I now feel more spiritual than physical. It is a case of constantly being in touch with your inner self, while drawing additional energy and information from your infinite soul. This should be a free-flowing exchange, but it will not work if someone else is directing you. In the past, I have had someone trying to intervene in this process, but it did not work. Your exchange needs to be pure and uncontaminated, where you will have a feeling, as in my case of 'a knowing', this being an act of love and for the benefit of your wellbeing, allowing the Universal energy to flow through you. When you let go of fear and negative energy, only then are you able to allow this vibration to enter your being and so attracting your aims and dreams into reality.

Only when you realise your helpers and guides are always with you, then you will never feel alone again. This perception has always been a source of great comfort to me.

Archangels have special responsibilities. For example, Michael for protecting yourself, your home, your family, if you are being attacked or if you are about to start a journey.

Archangel Raphael helps with healing, assists with your creativity and helps you achieve your goals, whereas

Gabriel has the responsibility for spirituality, love and hope.

If I feel disturbed at night and I feel I need protection, then I call on Archangel Michael to keep me safe. I then feel wings of feathers envelope me, making me feel safe and secure as I drift off to sleep. Also, when I ask for protection before embarking on a journey, I feel as if there is a vacuum surrounding my car, then I experience a trouble-free journey.

There is always a comforting feeling whenever I call upon the help of Archangel Michael. All anxieties seem to melt away, leaving me feeling more confident in the knowledge I am being protected.

I feel our guides are not always serious, but humorous too. I know I have one guide who is particularly jolly and he has often told me to be joyous too and not to worry so much. All is well and I need to trust.

It is interesting to observe, that no matter how much someone maybe in denial regarding their spirituality, every person calls on a higher power to help in times of great danger. Spirituality is fundamental to our very survival and so needs to be acknowledged and nurtured throughout our existence.

I believe we each need support from the universal Source, as being the very root of our existence. We live in our material world, being surrounded with objects, most of which are unnecessary but acquired to give us a false sense of security and self-worth. Looking more closely and deeper, this material reality changes into quantum reality, when all solid objects disappear because the atoms have no mass or size. Therefore, in quantum terms, the energy in an atom suggests the whole universe is vibrating at tremendous speeds which our senses are unable to visualise. Due to our senses being so slow, we are unable to register the frequency of vibrations, but instead, see solid objects.

One of my principal guides made himself known to me on my first day at University, when I was extremely apprehensive of my new venture, having spent the previous fourteen years at home raising my family. I remember feeling very anxious as I walked towards college, when for the first time, I heard my guide giving me encouragement, telling me I had far to go. (This statement actually came to fruition, after studying eight years at University and having a long career in Art and Design, with still lots more work to do today). My guide reassured me that all was well and I would receive constant support. This I became greatly aware of throughout my studies and career choice, particularly twelve years later, following a health scare, I was informed I must not worry about my mortality because I have much to do in this life and then my guide questioned, 'Have I ever told you untruths?' Ever since, I have erased any fear and focused instead on the job in hand, because I realise, I still have lots to do this time around.

Chapter 2

Miracles Do happen.

A wonderful example of how Spirit works in mysterious ways was during the early '60's, when Mike was in the army, being posted in Germany at the time. Once we became engaged, we saved hard for a year to raise the money to buy him out of the army, since he had a further six years to serve his full term. Our plan was for Mike to get a good job in the UK, buy a house and for us to get married.

While in Germany, Mike completed the obligatory application forms to buy himself out of the army and popped them in the post immediately. The very next day, Mike received 'posting orders' regarding his future postings to Borneo, Singapore and Hong Kong, all very premature since he had a further six months to serve in Germany. He was then told he was unable to now buy himself out because he was under 'posting orders'.

We were both devastated at this news because we were very much in love and wanted to be together, to settle in the UK, buying a home and getting married. (Some of those postings did not have married quarters, irrespective that I was now settled in a good job too).

This was the time I turned to Spirit for help, since we felt trapped in a situation which could change our lives. On the advice of Mike's Captain, someone he had befriended, he submitted an appeal. This Officer accompanied Mike to the tribunal, then acting on his behalf, stated that when the application to leave the army was posted to the UK, Mike was not aware of any future postings, no matter how premature. Even though the application was still in the post, not having yet arrived in the UK, on this technicality, thankfully, Mike was allowed to buy himself out of the army.

Needless to say, we were both very grateful for the intervention of the Captain and Spirit.

It seems that spirit is always around us in our daily lives. I know I have escaped death or serious injury on several occasions and yet miraculously survived. I was three years old when I was playing a ball game in a narrow alleyway with my best friend. The ball rolled away, down the path and onto a busy main road. Without a second thought, I swiftly ran after the ball and straight into the road, without looking, right into the path of a huge lorry. The driver had to struggle with an emergency stop, with only inches to spare before making contact with me. The driver was so shaken at the near disaster, he was in shock and he was taken into the nearby corner shop to recover. (The following year, my best friend made the same mistake, but she was not so fortunate).

It was years later, one dark evening I was coming out of the office, on my way home from work, when I almost fell down a large hole in the dark, directly outside the entrance of the building. There were no warning lights or cordons installed by the workmen. I miraculously jumped six feet, from a stationary position, tearing my skirt in the process. I still do not understand how I avoided an accident of falling down that deep hole.

There was another incident with a lorry, when I was visiting friends in Russia. I attempted to cross the road, forgetting to look in the opposite direction of the flow of traffic to that of the UK, when a lorry travelled at great speed past me. It was only the quick thinking of both my Russian friends who instinctively grabbed me by both arms and pulled me to safety, so thankfully a disaster was avoided.

One morning, I was visiting the supermarket, when I crossed the road to enter the store. Outside the shop was a red car, illegally parked on double yellow lines, with two ladies chatting inside. As I started to pass around the back of the vehicle, the driver reversed the car at speed, having used the wrong gear by mistake. As if by magic, I lurched the full width of the car, from standstill, arriving on the footpath. I still do not understand how I avoided being knocked over by the car. In fact, it was so close, a passing car braked, leaving the door wide open and the lady driver ran towards me since she had witnessed the incident and thought I was under the car. This lady was shocked and insisted I sat down for a while, but I felt fine, just a bit bewildered as to how I had avoided such a tragedy.

My husband used to be a fire-fighter when our children were small and one day, we were invited to a trip out, with a group of other work colleagues as a treat, onto a canal barge belonging to one of the firemen. As the boat glided into the mooring, at the end of our trip, I jumped onto the shrub and greenery on the towpath. However, unbeknown to me, there was no firm ground underneath, since the plants were overhanging the canal bank. Just as I was about to fall between the steel hull of the barge, as it drew into the metal of the canal side, a hand swiftly grabbed my shirt collar and hauled me back onto the barge. If it had not been for the swift action of one of the fire-fighters, I would have fallen and been squashed between the barge and the canal side. Once again, I realised I had narrowly avoided a tragedy.

On holiday in Chile, during the wintertime, I was at the bus station awaiting a bus to take us through the Andes into Argentina. I decided to visit the toilet before the long journey, since there were no toilets on board the bus. There was snow on the ground and the ladies toilets were down a very long flight of concrete steps. The floor was wet at the top of the stairs, due to the snow, when I slipped on the icy surface and started to fall down the stairs. I remember hitting the wall and banister a few times as I careered down the stairs, not once putting my feet on a step. I was aware of a youth sitting at a table at the foot of the stairs, waiting to take your money to use the toilets. He just sat with his mouth agape, as he saw the incident unfold. I ended up on both feet at the bottom of the stairs, very shaken but none the worse for wear. I felt I was definitely being helped down those steps, almost like magic.

To this day, I do not understand how or why I was saved, but I know I was assisted spiritually. They were miracles I experienced. It must not have been my time to pass and I believe we each have a path to follow during our time on earth and we do not go until our work is complete.

However, I try to keep my views private since I do not think it is our place to try to change the views of others and yet to balance this argument, I think it is important to pass on your knowledge while helping others understand.

There was a time, one of many, when I became aware of receiving help from spirit of some higher intelligence intervention. I was in my final year of my Honours Degree course at University, when each student had to exhibit their artwork, then for more than an hour, talk about your ideas and inspirations, followed by answering questions from fellow students, lecturers and other invited guests. I was extremely nervous about such a daunting task because I had no experience of public speaking and I knew there was some animosity and controversy about my work because of its realism and sublime spiritual content and so ahead of me was going to be a difficult time negotiating those tricky questions.

The Concourse was full of people awaiting my talk, far more than had attended other students' seminars and this just added to my anxiety, knowing rigorous questions were to follow for at least an hour. Most of my colleagues relied on alcohol to survive the ordeal, but I knew it was important to keep a clear head. However, I need not have worried. I meditated before I began my task, asking for help from my guides and then, just like magic, spirit took over. As the full concourse fell into silence, all faces pointing in my direction, I was amazed as I started talking with such confidence, that the time almost blurred, all questions articulately answered.

I was still in a trance-like state when I was congratulated regarding my performance. I am not sure how it happened, but I apparently talked eloquently for an hour, answering all their questions and yet I knew it was not 'me' who had been talking because someone else 'took over'. I do not know how I had navigated the difficult questions like a well-versed politician because I cannot remember what happened. I will never forget that experience but it just reinforced my belief that we are never alone. Help is there for everyone, if you only ask.

While understanding the importance of keeping an open mind, I read in the book, 'The Miracles of Archangel Michael' by Doreen Virtue, to ask Michael for protection if ever you found yourself in a fearful situation. Also, he was available to help you at any time, any place, even at the request to help others too. I have followed this advice many times and found it of a great help, if I am away from home and I wish my home to stay safe. This request is also useful for my family too since each of my adult children live many miles away. One son lives in Australia and so often, his home in the outback is at a risk to dreadful fires, due to the tinder dry grasses and gum-trees.

Three years ago, I was meditating when I asked Archangel Michael for protection of our family homes, that is the homes of my three adult children, my brother and our home too, while keeping our family safe. The time was approximately twelve noon.

I found out, just one hour later, that a huge gum tree had fallen, without warning towards my son's home in

Australia, with the top of the tree brushing the roof of his house. Fortunately, there was no structural damage to the house, but the metal seat my son had been sitting on that morning, while eating breakfast on the veranda, was completely flattened, so too the metal table, a metal water sculpture and also a strong metal pergola.

My son was very lucky that day because he sits there for all his meals in the summer. My daughter-in-law said the gum trees are called 'widow makers' because they fall without warning.

My son could have died that morning. Thank you, Archangel Michael.

Chapter 3

Orbs.

Within my family, we have photographic evidence of many orbs who are surrounding us, wherever we may go. On a trip to Egypt, we were able to photograph hundreds of orbs hovering in the night sky over the Temple at Luxor, during one evening as we sat on the boat, docked on the River Nile. At first, taken aback by the large quantity of orbs, we collected the same image using three different cameras. (See Figs 1&2).

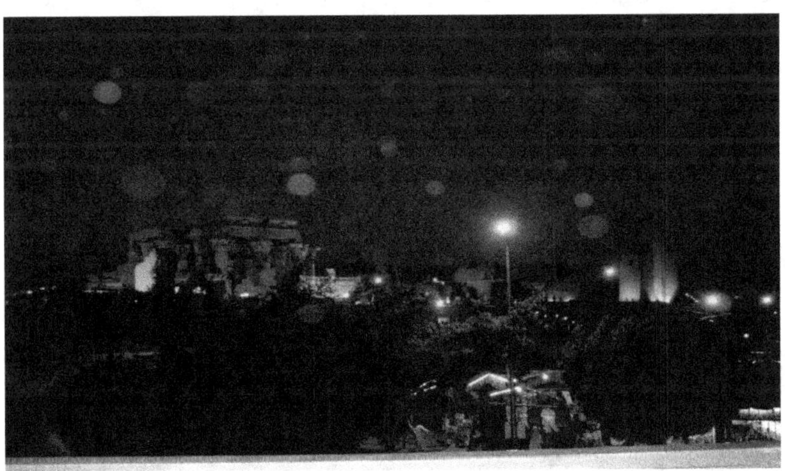

Fig 1 The Temple at Luxor, Egypt

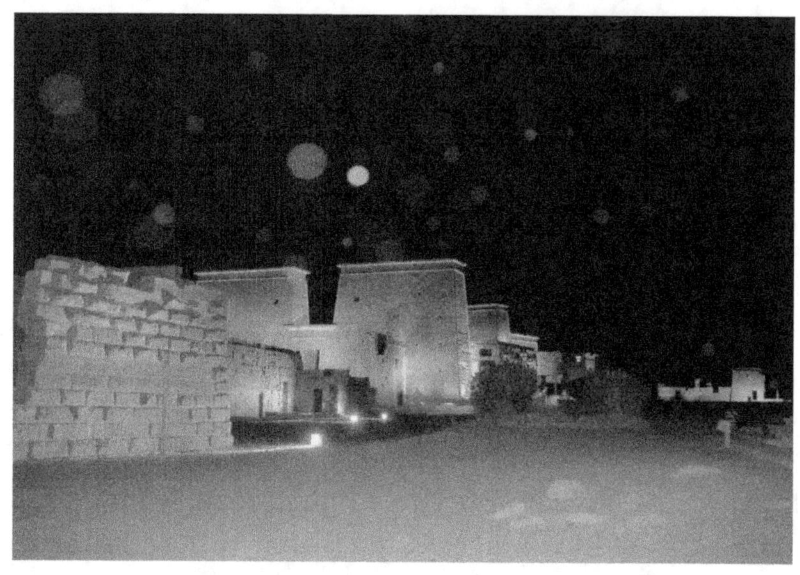

Fig 2. The Temple at Luxor, Egypt

There were many orbs inside the Egyptian Temples too. (See Figs 3&4).

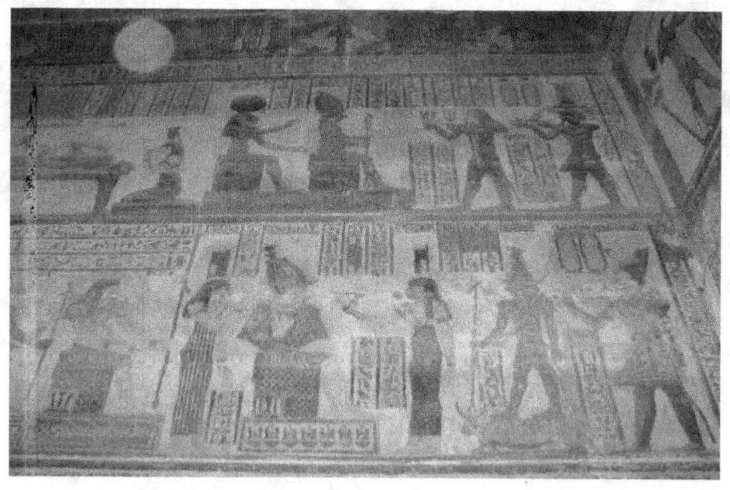

Fig 3 Inside Temple in Egypt.

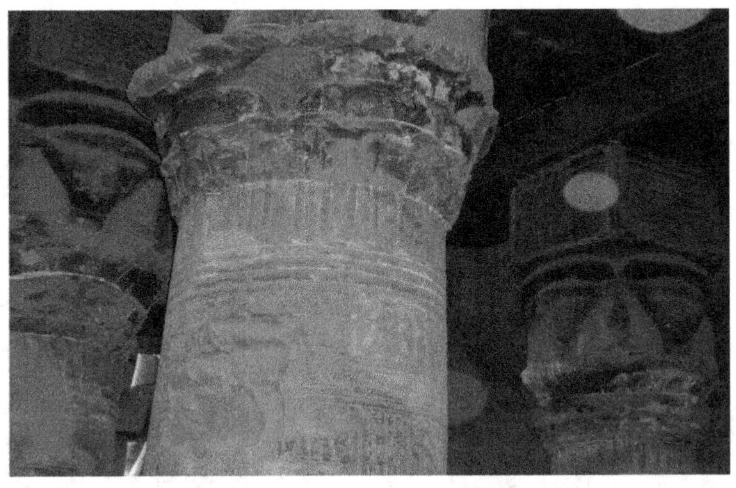

Fig 4 Inside Temple in Egypt.

On a visit to my son and his family in Australia, it was a rare occasion for our whole family to be together because our other son and daughter, together with her family in the UK, also joined us on this holiday. One day, we decided to go a lovely walk in the dense forest, with the narrow pathways cloaked in superb tree ferns. I then commented how wonderful if my parents were here too, even though they had passed away some years earlier. It was on our arrival in the U.K, we were looking at our photographs, when we noticed a few orbs within the forest. It was wonderful to know my parents had joined our family on this beautiful walk. (See Figs 5&6)

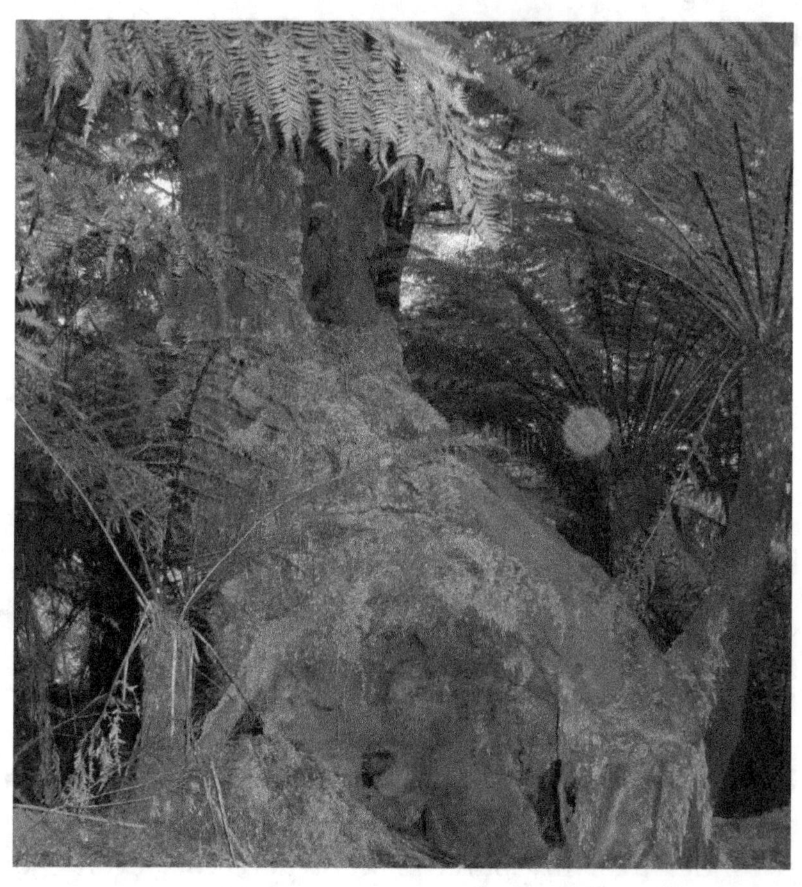

Fig 5 Inside the Australian fern forest.

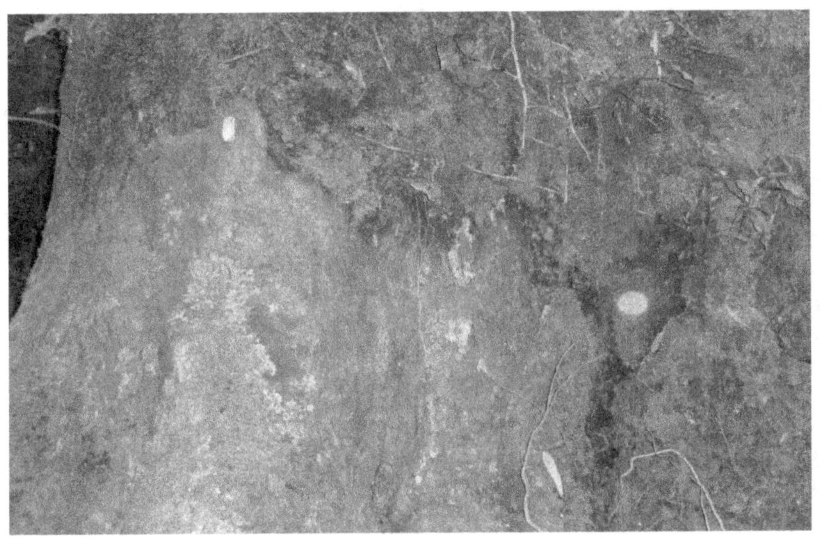

Fig 6 Inside the Australian fern forest.

During this particular holiday, we spent the Christmas holiday together too. When looking at photographs of my young grandson, opening his Christmas presents in the lounge, then on the leather sofa is yet another orb. (See Fig 7).

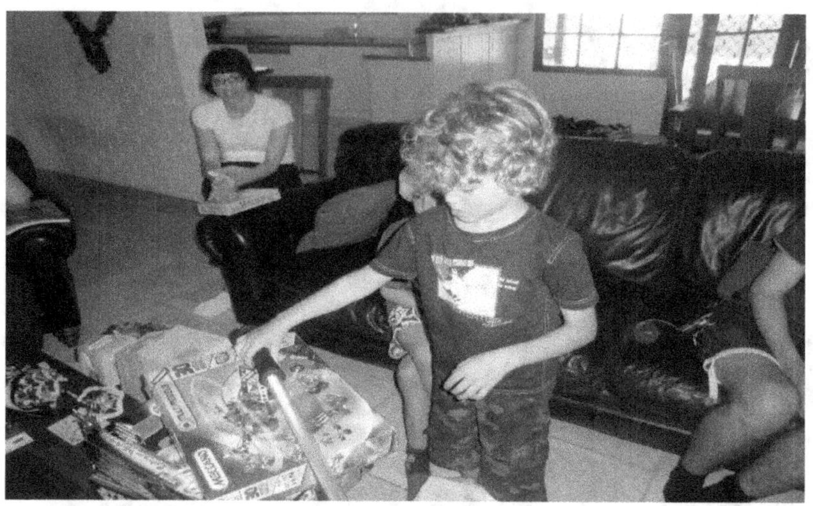

Fig 7 The Orb is on the sofa at Christmas in Australia.

This is confirmation that our loved ones are never far away, always joining in our activities, as if here on earth.

My grandson, who lives in England, was able to document orbs in France too, in particular around old abbeys, but we also have photographs of 'Willow the Wisp', my daughter aptly named the light swirls of smoke, frequently shown on photos around her young son. (See Fig 8).

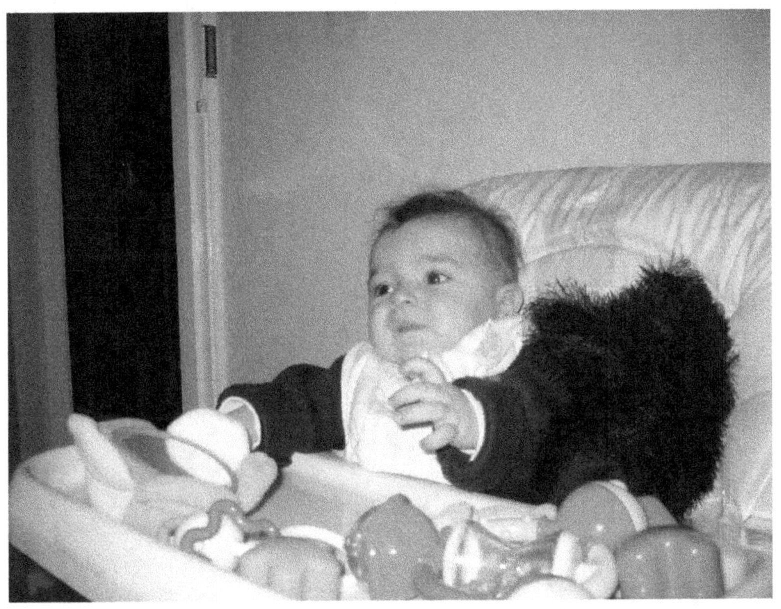

Fig 8 Joseph surrounded by 'Willow the Wisp'

Enlarging the photos of the orbs, some shine more brightly than others, while also of differing sizes and colours, yet there appears to be faces within some of the spheres too.

There is a book by Dr Klaus and Gundi Heinemann called 'Orbs: Their Mission and Messages of Hope', which includes many photographs of orbs, together with their in-depth research on the subject.

Chapter 4

When Helping Others,

We Are Helping Self.

I understand that I need to heal self, in order to be able to help other people. During the healing process, once I have made my intentions known to Spirit, regarding the healing, then I sort of step back while far more powerful Masters take over the procedure. It is as if I am a 'vehicle' to channel the healing energy.

When I have been aware of having a problem, then I have turned to meditation to ask for help and usually the right opportunity or person turns up in my life. In fact, for many years, I have always been on the lookout for meeting the 'right' person, or receiving a special invitation which maybe the key I have needed. Also, I specifically choose to live in a happy, peaceful place, stopping often during the day to remind myself to remain in this peaceful happy place, rather than being drawn into the lower energy fields of everyday dramas. It is a fact that if you are cheerful, then others respond. The vibrating energy between you lifts, to create a positive environment.

Whenever you see the Dali Lama being interviewed on the television, he is always smiling and often giggles, almost as if he has a private joke. One of my guides also laughs frequently, having a well-developed sense of humour and advised me not to take life too seriously, but to relax and have fun too.

It is a good idea to view all situations in your life and do not give energy to activities which no longer serve a purpose. Save it for the real things you desire in life. As with all successful people, stay focussed. making your intention known what you want, while asking for spiritual guidance along the way.

Another point Doreen Virtue mentions in her book, 'The Miracles of Archangel Michael', is about humans having invisible chords attached to our bodies and linking us to those people to whom we associate. (This is something I have been aware of when I refer to certain people as being 'energy suckers', those individuals who drain your energy). On your request, Archangel Michael will cut away any negative chords attached to your body, with his sword, freeing your energy while increasing your sense of wellbeing.

I have experienced this action and felt the remarkable benefits. I have also requested this help on a few occasions for another family member, whenever she is overwhelmed by a certain draining relationship in her life.

I am always open to try positive suggestions from different religions and philosophies, particularly where angels and saints are concerned.

Humans working through just the five senses do not appear to recognise that knowledge may be obtained intuitively, whereby with the multisensory experience, we are able to ask for help and receive instructions to aid our advancement. The five sensory humans only understand the power of learning through repetitive learning and techniques and yet there are also techniques available to learn intuitively.

If you work on yourself to clear any emotional blockages, then your vibrating frequency is heightened and so enables you to receive clear instructions. It is a case of constantly working on self to reduce any negativity, clearing away any anger at the end of each day, so you are able to operate on the level of unconditional love.

I believe only a section of our soul is incarnate in our body in this life on earth, maybe the part of the soul which needs to be healed or to have new experiences. I think when we request extra healing energy, we are tapping into our soul for extra reserves and in doing so, this additional pure energy invigorates and calms our body and mind. Although there is an endless supply for our needs, we receive a controlled amount so we are able to operate within the constraints of being in a human form.

Receiving instructions from not only our soul, but also from other guides, depending on their specialism, is of great comfort, to know there is an endless supply of loving support at our disposal. There is no such thing as loneliness, if only we realise, we are never alone. When our earthly life ends, we are then able to meet our helpers when we return home.

It is noticeable that the person who communicates on this level is more radiant and energetic than those who are working on a more physical level. You are operating on a spiritual, intuitive level within relationships, if you are caring, loving and concerned for the other person. When you are thinking of someone, other than yourself, then this is a deeper unconditional love. This is a more sincere, deeper love. However, if you are critical of another, concentrating on their faults, then this introduces negativity and conflict into the relationship.

As humans, we always seem to look outside ourselves for answers and yet if only we care to look within, all questions are answered. Almost all of my understanding of the world and relationships have come from my looking within, meditating and communicating with my guides and spiritual Masters. They are always ready to assist us with our perceptions of our world, to help us develop our intuition. As we are all connected in this vibrating mass, encompassing all living things in nature, we are all in this Universal energy together and so we need to love and help each other. When we are helping others, inadvertently, we are helping self.

If only everyone realised this profound statement, then all fear and negative actions would no longer exist. There would be no wars and we would live in harmony and peace. Everyone would be operating through unconditional love for each other and all living things.

However, much we may chase our desires, there will always be something we are unable to have, so it is much better for us to appreciate what we have already. If we count our blessings, then this will lead to contentment and happiness. His Holiness, the Dalai Lama, the spiritual leader of the Tibetan people talked about this subject, in the book, 'The Art of Happiness'

'The true antidote of greed is contentment. If you have a strong sense of contentment, it doesn't matter whether you obtain the object or not, either way, you are still content'.

It is a case of changing our thought patterns from negative into positive thoughts and in doing so, you are retraining your mind to be happy and content.

I believe our aim in life is to develop our spirit and bring it within our earthly body, then send out this 'Source love' to mankind. When this idea spreads, then the whole world will be living in harmony, according to God's law. I have not used the correct words to express myself, but I am getting the gist of the idea of living above the limited consciousness of earth, of being able to contact Source when meditating, just as if making a phone call.

Chapter 5

The Importance of Connecting

With Source.

I find it interesting to realise that we are able to recall our memory from many past years, through our thought process and yet this part of our brain is so small, it could not possibly hold so much information of facts and thoughts. This must occur outside our body, almost in a spiritual form. As I have mentioned earlier, I believe our soul is outside our physical body and it is a far greater part of us, than the small amount housed in our physical body. It is in this spiritual realm where we visit and receive guidance when we meditate. This is why it is important to take time out daily, to make contact with our guides within the spiritual domain.

Connecting with Source regularly is very important, whether it is helped through the sounds within music, feelings or meditation. It does not matter what method you use, just as long as you remember to continue with this practise. It will help keep you strong, centred and connected to your soul. If you do not practise regularly, then you will forget and so the benefits will be lost. The more the soul is contacted with love, compassion and empathy, then your vibration level increases to move ever closer to Source. Once we have this knowledge, then we need to start incorporating it in our everyday life.

Often people you meet are living their life out of fear or anger, but if only they re-connect to Source, in the knowledge they are not on their own, not separate but connected to each other and everyone, then there is no need for the feelings of insecurity.

Many of those insecurities may be acted out through the self-destructive addictions of drug abuse, alcoholism, self-harm, anorexia or obesity etc. All those negative activities are a plea for help, an attempt to distract from their feelings of isolation.

Remember, it is not necessary to look outwards for wisdom because we each have access within us, by contacting our soul energy to guide us. It is a good idea to have a special place in your home dedicated to your guides and teachers. For example, in my lounge I have made a spiritual place where I have candles, a statue of Buddha, a prayer plant and photos of my dear relatives who have passed over. This is where I light candles, burn incense and place fresh flowers in remembrance of those loved ones.

Although throughout our busy lives, we attract those people who draw on our energy, depleting our strength, it is important to regularly cut those emotional cords which often become attached by those needy people. By calling on Archangel Michael, he will use his sword to cut those negative cords, in order to set you free and yet he always allows the positive cords to remain. Archangel Michael and Archangel Raphael will both keep you safe and heal you, your energy field and aura, but do remember to thank them for looking after you, as expressing your gratitude is very important.

In her book, 'Seth Speaks', the metaphysical teacher Jane Roberts channels information from Seth regarding the truths that many of us have forgotten. We are reminded that we are far wiser than ever we imagined, even being more knowledgeable when we are dreaming. I know in the past I have solved some of my art problems while I have been asleep and Seth confirms our speech is much slower than our psychic communications, as we are informed or in receipt of information. This is something I have been aware of for years. To try to find the words to explain certain feelings and situations, speech is so laborious. This is because the physical self we recognise, works on a lower, slower vibration which is just a fragment of our total soul, since we each have a multidimensional personality, as infinite beings.

 I find I am frequently looking for someone to be able to teach me, on the physical plain but I have now realised my teachings have been those sent psychically from my guides and helpers, to assist me to connect with my inner identity. It is our own responsibility to find the Truth.

I believe the best wisdoms are gleaned from our guides, if only we remember to stop and listen. There may be a short while to wait because the guides maybe busy on other tasks, but I have found there are specialist in various areas too, e.g. artist, librarian, physician, oriental Reiki healer, general constant guide, angels and the Masters, all offering their assistance. There may be other close relatives too, who have now passed over the other side, who have our best interests at heart, while offering their support.

It is important to be secure in your sense of self, honour and spiritually centred, so your personal power is not eroded by external events, because losing power may lead to ill health.

An American author, Gary Paulsen, who commented that the busy city is a distraction and so when he enters the woods, his head clears and he feels calm.

'When you're on a sled behind a team, you enter
a state of primitive exultation, the solitude is
truly spiritual'.

I can so relate to this statement, having had a similar experience in the forest. Also:

'I'm running to something. I must have a
hundred ideas for books in my head.'

 I too have this same feeling of being driven, having nineteen projects still yet to be developed. As soon as I complete one idea, then two replace it, such is the power and enthusiasm for creativity.

On our spiritual journey it is possible to come into contact with negative forces at some time and so it is important to ask for protection, while keeping your energy high, so as not to be so vulnerable. As your energy raises, so does the protecting light.

In 1992, I was invited to visit a newly opened Gurdwara where I was fortunate to sit next to a Guru called Jiwan Singh Kalsa. At the time, I was having a problem with protecting myself from negative energy being emitted from other people. I asked the Guru for advice on how I could protect myself, when he told me to repeat the words, 'Satnam', meaning 'True Identity', or 'Wa he Guru', meaning 'Indescribable Wisdom'. It is important to use the correct words, rather than the translations because it is the vibrations of the original words which surround you with a field of protective energy. I have since used this method when I feel I need protection and it always works for me.

Early civilisations would gather in crowds to worship the sun at dawn. I remember my Mum telling me about one Easter-time, my Grandma took my Mum, who was just a young child at the time, out into the field at dawn, where they kept several horses. Just as the sun rose, that Easter morning, the horses, even her favourite horse, 'Poll,' knelt before the rising sun. I wonder if all animals do this every day? Maybe it is just that we are never there to witness this happening.

Chapter 6

Mike's Story.

Over the years, Mike had often asked how I could hear conversations from my guides. I used to tell him to keep practising meditation and eventually you will make contact with them. He is now proficient with this method of communication and when we both heal in silence, we compare notes afterwards and the guides present, activities and conversations during the healing times, are exactly the same for each of us.

In 1995, Mike was sent to the USA for a month, on business. On his return, I was very surprised to be presented with a long-written account of his spiritual encounter, (something Mike had never attempted before or since), so profound was his experience.

During his meditation session while away, when resting in bed at the end of the day, he became aware of a Master spirit guide who told him to sit up in bed. Well, Mike has always found this task very difficult because he has a genetic problem of four fused vertebrae in his spine, so sitting up in bed is extremely difficult for him. He spoke out to say he was unable to do this, when the voice told him he would be fine. Mike, fully awake by this time, sat up in bed with ease. He was then told he would be able to look through a book of his past lives. At first the pages of the book turned slowly, showing scenes as if watching video clips of Sioux Indians hunting buffalo on the North American plains. This was a time before horses had been introduced to the tribes and Mike was with his friends hunting the buffalo with spears, bow and arrows. There were a number of dead animals, when one wounded buffalo turned and charged towards Mike, who tried to hide behind a dead animal. Alas, he was not quick enough and so he was hit in the middle of his back. The next scene was where Mike was lying on the ground, surrounded by his tribe, as he slipped away. He was told by the Master spirit guide that the persistent back problem was as a result of his broken back accident with the charging buffalo.

The next page showed him in another life as an old Indian, being laid down in the snow to die, because he was unable to keep up with the moving tribe. Even now, he feels alright with this behaviour because it was the Sioux way.

The third life as a North American Indian was as a young man who had been out hunting with his friends, when he returned to his tepee being on fire, with his wife and child still inside. He tried to rescue them but was held back because his family were already dead inside the tent. I might add that Mike remembers a lot of information regarding his life and customs of his time as a Sioux Indian.

The following pages of the book showed Mike as an Aztec or Mayan warrior with black and yellow paint on his body and black and yellow plumes in his hair.

Many previous times as a North American Indian on the prairies, being given descriptions and information of his names and those of his wives, children, friends, various deaths, then walking through the mist into other past lives. Mike was shown times when he lived in different cultures, the pace quickening as he progressed through numerous lives, but not in the chronological sequence as we know them. There were just glimpses of being male and yet other times, female too and then the pages reduced speed as he was shown his last life, as a soldier in a Tank Regiment during World War 11, prior to this present time.

Before returning to the UK, Mike tried to make contact on another occasion but was told to think about his journey and to find some answers.
On his arrival home, Mike was very moved by his experience in USA, in particular with regard to the three lives he remembered as a North American Indian, a time when he was very happy and close with nature. He still retains such a deep connection with that culture and treasured memories of those times into his present lifetime.

It was four years later, following a disastrous affair, when Mike and I almost divorced, that his story continues.

One night, in late 1999, I awoke in the early hours and started to meditate, expressing gratitude that Mike was now 'safely back home' because he nearly did not make it. There were evil forces involved, trying to take him away.

I became aware of a great Master being present when I was guided to start the process of 'cleaning' Mike's body, as he slept. There was so much crackling energy, as I set to work, scanning his body with this negative energy bouncing off my hand, off my wrist and up my arm. This was the first time I had experienced something so disturbing. It was very alarming.

As the cleansing continued and Mike's aura began feeling more neutral, I then became aware of there now being two great Masters present, both of the same high rank, who were great friends in the spirit world, even though they were from different cultures. As I asked for protection for each member of our family, since we were vulnerable to this evil, Mike then began to stir from his sleep. I whispered he was now safe, to reassure him, since he had been on a very dangerous journey. I was then startled when Mike started to talk slowly and deeply, not his usual pitch of voice but that deliberate tone as if he was a North American Indian. He continued with this long conversation with me, as if he was under hypnosis.

I explained I had seen the great spirit White Eagle and commenced describing him as a strong, proud man, with a turned down mouth and a deliberate, slow speech. Mike confirmed my description and commented that White Eagle was a very good spirit, a good warrior on the other side too. Mike said he had been on a very dangerous journey where he had been tricked by evil forces. Everything started to go wrong a year earlier, when he was in mourning for 'Morning Dove and Little Bird', (his wife and daughter during one of his Indian life-times, who were burned in a tepee fire). He decided to leave his tepee and family, to go on his quest to find 'Morning Dove and Little Bird'. He left his best friend, Black Fox, in charge of us while he, Running Buffalo, set on his travels.

When he tried to contact White Eagle, there was lots of mist so he could not see him but he could hear direction. Only now does Mike, as Running Buffalo, know it was evil spirits hiding in the mist, taking on the identity of White Eagle.

This is when Mike, mistakenly thought a work colleague and her daughter were 'Morning Dove and little Bird'. (It was at this moment when White Eagle interrupted the session to say the real 'Morning Dove' is actually our daughter in this present lifetime).

Mike continued his conversation by saying he did not realise he was being tricked and went through great torment, so much so that the evil spirits almost killed him.

Only now does Mike realise what great love our current family have for him and that he knows his job is to stay in the tepee to protect us. He said it will never, ever happen again and that he has staked himself down in the tepee so he can never wander again.

White Eagle then said I had been a good warrior to protect Mike and that I was a bright beacon within the family. Our children are very strong, with good spirits, so when the time comes, they will lead others to safety, because soon there will be a black time, but good will win over evil.

At the moment, there are lots of evil spirits around looking for victims and Mike was lured away because they wanted to get into his tepee to mortally wound his family. However, he is back with us now and it will not happen again. He is so happy to be back home and he is here to protect us.

I asked White Eagle when did Mike make the decision to return home.
He said Mike was still in turmoil when driving home on the motorway, but then the real White Eagle spoke to him clearly, the mist had now cleared by this time and Mike knew it was the true White Eagle who advised him to return home to us.

White Eagle then continued to explain that Mike had been on a very dangerous journey and he had learned many things but he was very tired now and so needed to rest.

Mike then stopped talking in this hypnotic state and fell asleep. I also slept, while making a mental note to record this incident on waking, since this was a new experience for me, making contact with White Eagle, the whole story and meditation, with Mike speaking in a hypnotic state, sounding as a North American Indian.

The next morning, I wrote my account at 6.30am, as Mike slept heavily, as if exhausted. I now understand why our daughter took an instant dislike to this impersonator. She was rather very angry and repulsed that this person should be in our home.

On waking, Mike remembered nothing of the conversations, but this incident has made a clear impression on us both, up to this present day, such is the rich tapestry of life.

I realise that the most important point of my aim is to help heal someone else, even though I may not have the knowledge. It is your intention that has the healing effect, through the Source energy, a knowing and trust in the knowledge that healing will follow. Usually, it is those who have a strong spiritual belief and who belong to a close network of family and friends who tend to live much longer too and the more I contemplate on the subject, I realise there is so much more for us to learn about the all-encompassing power of the universal energy. It is almost operating similar to a vast communications computer, relaying constant messages through energy waves to each of us, in an attempt to support and help us understand our place in this swirling cosmic soup.

www.ingramcontent.com/pod-product-compliance
Lightning Source LLC
Chambersburg PA
CBHW061739250726
48657CB00002B/1010